# DASH DIET FOR HEART HEALTH

A Heart Health and Kidney Function Improvement Program Based on America's Top-Rated Diet with Tasty and Delicious Recipes to Lower Blood Pressure Together. (2-in-1 Book)

**Thomas Moore Clay**

# ABOUT THE AUTHOR

*Thomas Moore Clay is a distinguished and compassionate nutritionist and dietician who has dedicated his life to transforming the health and well-being of countless individuals. With an unwavering commitment to improving the lives of his clients, he has become a renowned figure in the field of nutrition and health management, with a particular focus on addressing the pervasive issue of high blood pressure.*

*With an extensive educational background in nutrition and dietetics, Thomas Moore Clay possesses a deep understanding of the intricate relationship between diet and overall health. He has channeled this knowledge into a successful career marked by numerous achievements and a remarkable track record of helping those in need.*

*Over the years, Thomas Moore Clay has made a significant impact on the lives of over 300 individuals battling health problems, particularly high blood pressure. His approach goes beyond just offering dietary advice; he provides personalized, holistic solutions that address the root causes of his clients' health issues. His dedication to improving their quality of life is truly unparalleled.*

*Thomas Moore Clay's work extends far beyond the consultation room. He is a strong advocate for healthy living, regularly sharing his expertise through public speaking engagements, workshops, and educational initiatives. His mission is not only to help individuals regain control over their health but also to empower them with the knowledge and tools to sustain a healthier lifestyle.*

*With a heart full of compassion and a mind brimming with knowledge, Thomas Moore Clay has become a trusted name in the field of nutrition and dietetics. His impact on the health and well-being of so many is a testament to his unwavering commitment to making the world a healthier place, one person at a time.*

# TABLE OF CONTENTS

# INTRODUCTION

In the small, vibrant town of Greenwood, Sarah, a 42-year-old elementary school teacher, faced a turning point in her life. Known for her contagious smile and boundless energy, Sarah's life took an unexpected turn during a routine health check-up. Her doctor voiced concerns about her elevated blood pressure and cholesterol levels, words that echoed in her mind: "risk of heart disease." It was a wake-up call for Sarah, who had a family history of heart conditions. Determined to rewrite her health story, she embarked on a journey that led her to the DASH Diet, a path that not only transformed her health but also gave her a new lease on life.

## What is the DASH Diet?

DASH, which stands for Dietary Approaches to Stop Hypertension, is more than just a diet; it's a lifelong approach to healthy eating designed to help treat or prevent high blood pressure (hypertension). The DASH Diet encourages reducing sodium intake and eating a variety of nutrient-rich foods that help lower blood pressure, such as potassium, calcium, and magnesium.

For Sarah, the DASH Diet was not just about following a set of dietary rules; it was about embarking on a journey towards a healthier heart. She learned that the diet focuses on fruits, vegetables, whole grains, and lean proteins, while limiting foods high in saturated fat, sugar, and sodium. The emphasis on fresh, unprocessed food was a shift from her previous eating habits, which often included convenient but unhealthy choices.

## Origins and Development

The origins of the DASH Diet date back to the early 1990s when the National Institutes of Health (NIH) funded research to explore the effects of dietary patterns on blood pressure. The landmark DASH study emerged, showing that a diet rich in fruits, vegetables, and low-fat dairy foods, with reduced saturated and total fat, could substantially lower blood pressure. It wasn't designed as a weight-loss program; it was a formula for heart health, a fact that resonated with Sarah as she learned more about the diet's background.

Subsequent studies reinforced these findings and expanded our understanding of the diet's benefits, including its role in lowering cholesterol, managing diabetes, and even assisting with weight management. This body of research provided Sarah with the confidence that she was on the right path.

## Principles of the DASH Diet

**Emphasis on Whole Foods:** The diet focuses on whole, unprocessed foods, a stark contrast to the high-sodium, preservative-laden foods that are common in many diets. This principle guided Sarah to make healthier food choices, like opting for fresh fruits instead of sugary snacks.

**Rich in Fruits and Vegetables:** These are the cornerstones of the DASH Diet. They're not only low in calories but are also rich sources of essential nutrients and fiber. Sarah found that incorporating a variety of colors and types of fruits and vegetables made her meals more enjoyable and satisfying.

**Inclusion of Whole Grains:** The diet encourages whole grains over refined grains. Sarah learned to love brown rice, whole wheat bread, and quinoa, appreciating their role in heart health.

**Lean Proteins and Low-Fat Dairy:** The diet suggests moderate amounts of lean protein and low-fat or non-fat dairy. Sarah discovered the versatility of lean meats like chicken and fish and embraced dairy alternatives like almond milk.

**Limited Sodium, Saturated Fats, and Sugars:** Reducing sodium intake is a crucial aspect of the DASH Diet. Sarah became vigilant about reading food labels, surprised by the high sodium content in many packaged foods. She also limited her intake of saturated fats and added sugars, which are known to adversely affect heart health.

**Balance and Moderation:** The DASH Diet is not about strict rules or deprivation but about balance and moderation. It allowed Sarah the flexibility to enjoy her favorite foods in moderation, making the diet sustainable in the long term.

Through her journey, Sarah realized that the DASH Diet was more than a set of dietary guidelines; it was a catalyst for a healthier lifestyle. She started pairing her new eating habits with regular exercise, initially with brisk walks, and then gradually incorporating more activities like yoga and cycling.

The transformation was remarkable. Within months, Sarah's energy levels soared, her blood pressure normalized, and her cholesterol levels improved significantly. But more than the physical benefits, it was the sense of empowerment and control over her health that truly changed her life.

Sarah's story is a testament to the power of the DASH Diet as a tool for heart health. It's not just a diet; it's a holistic approach to a healthier, happier life. As she often shares with her friends and family, "It's not about the restrictions; it's about making smarter choices and enjoying the journey towards a healthier heart."

# Part I
# Understanding
# Heart Health

# CHAPTER 1

# THE HEART: AN OVERVIEW

The heart is an extraordinary organ, central to our very existence. Understanding its anatomy, the common diseases that afflict it, and the risk factors associated with heart disease is crucial for anyone interested in maintaining cardiovascular health.

## Anatomy and Function of the Heart

The heart, an organ about the size of a clenched fist, is not just central to the human body but to the very essence of life. Tucked away in the chest, slightly to the left of center, it serves as the powerhouse of the cardiovascular system. This muscular organ's primary role is to pump blood throughout the body, ensuring the delivery of oxygen and essential nutrients to various tissues while simultaneously removing metabolic waste products like carbon dioxide.

### Detailed Structure of the Heart

Understanding the heart's anatomy is key to appreciating its complex functionality. The heart is divided into four distinct chambers: the left and right atria (upper chambers) and the left and right ventricles (lower chambers). Each of these chambers plays a crucial role in the heart's circulatory process.

- **Atria:** The atria are the smaller, upper chambers of the heart. Their primary function is to receive blood. The right atrium receives deoxygenated blood from the body, while the left atrium receives oxygenated blood from the lungs. These chambers act as reservoirs, preparing to send blood into the ventricles.

- **Ventricles:** The ventricles are the larger, more muscular lower chambers. They are the main pumping chambers of the heart. The right ventricle pumps the deoxygenated blood it receives from the right atrium to the lungs for oxygenation, while the left ventricle pumps oxygenated blood to the rest of the body.

- **Valves:** The heart contains four vital valves – the tricuspid, pulmonary, mitral, and aortic valves. The tricuspid valve is located between the right atrium and right ventricle, and the pulmonary valve is between the right ventricle and the pulmonary artery. On the left side of the heart, the mitral valve separates the left atrium and left ventricle, and the aortic valve is between the left ventricle and the aorta. These valves act as one-way gates, ensuring that blood flows in the correct direction and preventing backflow.

- **Septum:** The septum is a wall of muscle that separates the left and right sides of the heart. It is crucial in ensuring that oxygenated and deoxygenated blood do not mix.

## Circulation Process

The heart's primary role in circulation can be divided into two main pathways: the systemic and pulmonary circuits.

- **Pulmonary Circuit:** This involves the movement of blood between the heart and the lungs. It begins when deoxygenated blood from the body flows into the right atrium, moves into the right ventricle, and is then pumped through the pulmonary artery to the lungs. In the lungs, carbon dioxide is exchanged for oxygen, transforming the blood into oxygen-rich blood.

- **Systemic Circuit:** Oxygen-rich blood then travels back to the heart, entering the left atrium, then the left ventricle. From here, it is pumped through the aorta and distributed throughout the body via a network of arteries, arterioles, and capillaries. This oxygenated blood provides essential nutrients and oxygen to body tissues, and after the exchange, the now deoxygenated blood returns to the heart through veins, completing the cycle.

**Electrical System of the Heart**

The heart's functionality is not only mechanical but also electrical. Its electrical system is what controls the rate and rhythm of the heartbeat.

- **Sinoatrial (SA) Node:** Often referred to as the heart's natural pacemaker, the SA node is located in the right atrium. It generates electrical impulses that initiate each heartbeat. These impulses cause the atria to contract, pushing blood into the ventricles.

- **Atrioventricular (AV) Node:** The impulses from the SA node then travel to the AV node, located between the atria and ventricles. There's a slight delay at the AV node, allowing the ventricles time to fill with blood from the atria.

- **Conduction Pathways:** From the AV node, the impulses travel along a path of specialized cells in the walls of the ventricles, causing them to contract. This contraction propels the blood out of the heart – to the lungs from the right ventricle and to the body from the left ventricle.

This electrical system ensures that the heart beats in a coordinated and rhythmic manner, typically around 60 to 100 times per minute at rest. It's this precise coordination that allows the heart to function effectively as a pump.

**Significance of Heart Function**

The heart's role extends beyond its mechanical and electrical functions. It is integral to the overall well-being of the body. The efficiency of the heart's pumping action affects the delivery of nutrients and oxygen to tissues, the removal of waste products, and the maintenance of blood pressure. Any disruption in its function can have widespread effects on overall health.

# Common Heart Diseases

Heart diseases, collectively known as cardiovascular diseases, are a significant health concern worldwide. They encompass a range of conditions that affect the heart's structure and function, each with its unique characteristics and implications. Understanding these common heart diseases is crucial for early detection, effective management, and prevention.

## 1. Coronary Artery Disease (CAD)

Coronary Artery Disease is the most prevalent form of heart disease. It occurs when the coronary arteries, responsible for supplying blood to the heart muscle, become hardened and narrowed. This condition, known as atherosclerosis, is caused by the buildup of plaque, a mixture of fat, cholesterol, calcium, and other substances found in the blood. Over time, this buildup can restrict or even completely block blood flow to the heart muscle.

*Symptoms and Complications:* The reduced blood flow can lead to chest pain or discomfort known as angina, one of the most common symptoms of CAD. In more severe cases, it can cause a heart attack, where part of the heart muscle is starved of oxygen and begins to die.

This is a medical emergency and requires immediate treatment.

***Risk Factors:*** Risk factors for CAD include high blood pressure, high cholesterol levels, smoking, diabetes, obesity, physical inactivity, and a family history of heart disease. Lifestyle changes and medications can effectively manage and reduce these risks.

## 2. Heart Failure

Heart failure, often misunderstood as the heart stopping, is a condition where the heart doesn't pump blood as efficiently as it should. This inefficiency can be due to the heart's inability to fill with enough blood (diastolic heart failure) or its inability to pump with sufficient force (systolic heart failure).

***Causes and Symptoms:*** The most common causes of heart failure include coronary artery disease, high blood pressure, and cardiomyopathy. Symptoms of heart failure include shortness of breath, fatigue, swollen legs, and rapid heartbeat. Managing heart failure involves treating the underlying cause, lifestyle changes, and medications to improve heart function and relieve symptoms.

# 3. Arrhythmias

Arrhythmias refer to any irregularity in the heart's rhythm. They can manifest as tachycardia (a heart rate that's too fast), bradycardia (a heart rate that's too slow), or irregular heartbeat.

***Types and Effects:*** Common types of arrhythmias include atrial fibrillation, where the upper chambers of the heart beat irregularly and out of coordination with the lower chambers, and ventricular fibrillation, a life-threatening condition where the heart's lower chambers quiver and cannot pump blood. Symptoms can range from a fluttering in the chest to fainting, and they can increase the risk of stroke or heart failure. Treatment varies based on the type and severity of the arrhythmia but may include medications, lifestyle changes, or procedures like pacemaker implantation.

# 4. Valvular Heart Disease

Valvular heart disease is characterized by damage to or a defect in one of the four heart valves: the mitral, aortic, tricuspid, or pulmonary valves. These valves regulate blood flow through the heart.

***Types and Treatments:*** Common types of valvular disease include stenosis (narrowing of the valve), regurgitation (leakage of the valve), and atresia (a valve that isn't properly formed). Symptoms depend on which valve is affected but can include shortness of breath, fatigue, irregular heartbeat, swollen feet or ankles, and chest pain. Treatment may involve medication, lifestyle changes, or surgery to repair or replace the affected valve.

## 5. Cardiomyopathy

Cardiomyopathy refers to diseases of the heart muscle. In cardiomyopathy, the heart muscle becomes enlarged, thick, or rigid, impairing its ability to pump blood effectively. In some cases, the heart muscle tissue is replaced with scar tissue.

***Forms and Consequences:*** There are several forms of cardiomyopathy, including dilated, hypertrophic, and restrictive cardiomyopathy. The condition can lead to heart failure, arrhythmias, and sudden cardiac death. Symptoms may include breathlessness, swelling in the legs and abdomen, fatigue, and palpitations. Treatments focus on managing symptoms, slowing the disease's progression, and reducing the risk of complications. This may include lifestyle changes, medications, and in some cases, devices like pacemakers or defibrillators, or heart transplant in advanced stages.

## Risk Factors for Heart Disease

Understanding the risk factors for heart disease is crucial in its prevention and management. These factors can be categorized into modifiable (those you can change) and non-modifiable (those you cannot change).

**Modifiable Risk Factors:**

- **Unhealthy Diet:** A diet high in saturated fats, trans fats, sodium, and cholesterol has been linked to heart disease and related conditions, like hypertension and atherosclerosis.

- **Physical Inactivity:** Lack of regular physical activity can contribute to poor heart health and is a major risk factor for heart disease.

- **Obesity:** Excess body weight, especially around the waist, increases the risk of heart disease.

- **Excessive Alcohol Use:** Heavy drinking can lead to increased blood pressure, heart failure, and stroke.

- **Smoking:** Smoking damages the blood vessels and can lead to heart disease.

- **High Blood Pressure (Hypertension):** This increases the heart's workload, causing the heart muscle to thicken and become stiffer.

- **High Cholesterol:** High levels of bad cholesterol (LDL) can lead to the buildup of plaques in the arteries, increasing the risk of heart attack and stroke.

**Non-Modifiable Risk Factors:**

- **Age:** The risk of heart disease increases with age.

- **Gender:** Men are generally at greater risk of heart disease, though the risk for women increases after menopause.

- **Family History:** A family history of heart disease increases your risk, especially if a parent developed it at an early age.

- **Ethnicity:** Certain ethnic groups are at higher risk for heart disease. For instance, African Americans are more likely to have high blood pressure and heart disease.

- **Pre-existing Health Conditions:** Conditions like diabetes can increase the risk of heart disease.

# CHAPTER 2

# NUTRITION AND HEART HEALTH

## The Role of Diet in Heart Health

Understanding the role of diet in heart health is akin to comprehending how the quality of fuel impacts the performance and longevity of an engine. In this analogy, our heart is the engine, and our diet is the fuel. The quality of this fuel – what we consume – directly influences not only the efficiency of our heart but also its longevity and strength. This relationship between our dietary choices and heart health encompasses more than just avoiding harmful foods; it involves an active selection of foods that promote cardiovascular strength and endurance.

### The Power of Whole Foods

Whole foods – fruits, vegetables, whole grains, lean proteins, and healthy fats – are the stalwarts of heart health. These foods are treasure troves of essential nutrients, fiber, and antioxidants, each playing a crucial role in supporting the heart's functions.

- **Fruits and Vegetables: Nature's Heart Protectors**

Fruits and vegetables are vital in regulating blood pressure and preventing arterial damage. Rich in vitamins and minerals, they help in maintaining electrolyte balance, crucial for heart function. The fiber in fruits and vegetables also plays a significant role in heart health. Soluble fiber, found in foods like apples, berries, and oats, helps lower low-density lipoprotein (LDL) or 'bad' cholesterol, a known contributor to heart disease. Additionally, the antioxidants in fruits and vegetables, such as flavonoids and beta-carotene, protect the heart by reducing oxidative stress and inflammation, which can damage heart vessels and tissues.

- **Whole Grains: Sustained Energy and Vascular Health**

Whole grains are integral to a heart-healthy diet. Unlike refined grains, whole grains retain all parts of the grain kernel, including the bran, germ, and endosperm, which are rich in nutrients. Consuming whole grains like brown rice, quinoa, and whole wheat helps in maintaining a healthy weight, thereby reducing the risk of heart disease. They are also high in dietary fiber, which helps to lower cholesterol levels and stabilize blood sugar levels, preventing spikes and crashes that can stress the heart.

- **Lean Proteins: Building Blocks for a Healthy Heart**
Lean proteins, including fish, poultry, legumes, and plant-based proteins, provide essential amino acids without the excess saturated fats found in higher-fat meat products. Fatty fish such as salmon, mackerel, and sardines are especially beneficial due to their high omega-3 fatty acid content. These fats are known for their anti-inflammatory properties and their ability to reduce triglycerides, lower blood pressure, and decrease the risk of arrhythmias. Plant-based proteins like lentils, beans, and tofu are not only good sources of protein but also contain fiber and various phytonutrients, contributing further to heart health.

- **Healthy Fats: Essential Yet Misunderstood**
Healthy fats, particularly mono- and polyunsaturated fats, are crucial for heart health. Sources include olive oil, avocados, nuts, and seeds. These fats help in reducing the levels of harmful LDL cholesterol and increasing the levels

of beneficial high-density lipoprotein (HDL) cholesterol. They also aid in the absorption of fat-soluble vitamins, which are essential for various bodily functions, including those of the heart.

**Limiting Harmful Foods**

Conversely, certain types of foods pose significant risks to heart health and should be consumed in moderation or avoided.

- **The Dangers of Trans and Saturated Fats**
  Trans fats, often found in fried and baked goods, and saturated fats, prevalent in fatty meats and dairy products, can increase LDL cholesterol levels. These fats contribute to the formation of plaques in the arteries, a condition known as atherosclerosis, which can lead to heart attacks and strokes. Limiting the intake of these fats is crucial for maintaining a healthy heart.

- **Sodium: A Stealthy Culprit**
  Sodium, commonly consumed in excess through processed and fast foods, can contribute to high blood pressure, a major risk factor for heart disease. Excess sodium intake causes the body to

retain water, putting extra pressure on the heart
and blood vessels.

- **The Impact of Sugars and Refined Carbohydrates**

  Sugary foods and beverages, along with refined carbohydrates, are major contributors to obesity, a significant risk factor for heart disease. These foods can lead to rapid spikes in blood sugar and insulin levels, contributing to inflammation, high blood pressure, and eventually, to the wear and tear of the cardiovascular system.

## Nutrients Essential for a Healthy Heart

The quest for heart health is deeply rooted in the nutrients we consume. A heart-healthy diet is rich in specific nutrients that play crucial roles in maintaining cardiovascular health. Understanding and incorporating these nutrients into our daily diet can significantly enhance heart function and reduce the risk of heart diseases. Let's delve deeper into these essential nutrients.

**Fiber: The Heart's Ally**

Fiber, found in abundance in fruits, vegetables, and whole grains, is a formidable ally for heart health. It's not just about aiding digestion; fiber plays a pivotal role in cholesterol management. Soluble fiber, found in foods like oats, apples, and beans, dissolves in water to form a gel-like substance in the digestive tract. This substance binds with cholesterol particles and aids in their excretion from the body. By reducing the absorption of cholesterol into the bloodstream, soluble fiber effectively lowers the levels of low-density lipoprotein (LDL), commonly known as 'bad' cholesterol.

Moreover, fiber-rich diets are associated with a lower risk of developing heart diseases. They contribute to weight management, as high-fiber foods are more filling and can reduce overall calorie intake. This is crucial because obesity is a significant risk factor for heart disease.

**Omega-3 Fatty Acids: The Anti-Inflammatory Powerhouses**

Omega-3 fatty acids, primarily found in fatty fish like salmon, mackerel, and sardines, as well as in flaxseeds and walnuts, are celebrated for their cardiovascular benefits. These fats are essential, meaning the body cannot produce them, and they must be obtained through diet. Their anti-inflammatory properties are critical in reducing the inflammation that can damage blood vessels and lead to heart disease.

Omega-3s play a significant role in lowering triglyceride levels in the blood. High levels of triglycerides, a type of fat, are linked to an increased risk of coronary artery disease. These fatty acids also help in reducing blood pressure, a major risk factor for heart disease. Furthermore, omega-3 fatty acids are known to decrease the risk of arrhythmias - irregular heartbeats that can lead to sudden death. They also improve endothelial function, which is the health of the lining of the blood vessels, and reduce blood clotting, thus decreasing the risk of heart attacks and strokes.

**Antioxidants: The Protectors of the Heart**

Antioxidants, including vitamins C and E, play a significant role in protecting the heart. Found in a variety of fruits and vegetables, these powerful substances combat free radicals - unstable molecules that can cause oxidative stress, leading to damage of the blood vessels and other tissues.

Vitamin C, abundant in citrus fruits, strawberries, bell peppers, and broccoli, enhances the body's ability to repair damaged tissues and reduces the risk of cardiovascular disease. Vitamin E, found in nuts, seeds, and vegetable oils, helps protect against the oxidation of LDL cholesterol, a key factor in the development of atherosclerosis (hardening of the arteries). Together, these antioxidants help in maintaining the structural integrity of the blood vessels and prevent various forms of heart disease.

## Potassium: The Balancing Mineral

Potassium, a mineral found in foods like bananas, oranges, potatoes, and spinach, is essential for maintaining a healthy blood pressure level. It works in opposition to sodium to maintain fluid balance in the body and help relax blood vessel walls, which aids in reducing blood pressure. High blood pressure is a significant risk factor for heart disease, including heart attacks and strokes.

Potassium also plays a role in heart muscle function, including the rhythmic contractions of the heart. A diet rich in potassium can help regulate heart rate and ensure smooth and coordinated heart muscle contractions, essential for maintaining a healthy heart rhythm.

**Magnesium and Calcium: The Dynamic Duo for Heart Muscle Function**

Magnesium and calcium, two minerals essential for heart health, are found in dairy products, leafy greens, nuts, and seeds. These minerals work in concert to support heart muscle function and blood pressure regulation.

Magnesium acts as a natural calcium channel blocker, a type of medication often prescribed to lower blood pressure. It helps relax and widen blood vessels, making it easier for the heart to pump blood. Moreover, magnesium is involved in over 300 biochemical reactions in the body, including energy production and muscle contraction, making it vital for overall heart health.

Calcium, on the other hand, is essential for the proper contraction of the heart muscle. It plays a critical role in the electrical conduction system of the heart, ensuring that the heart beats properly. A balanced intake of calcium, in conjunction with magnesium, is crucial in maintaining a healthy heart rhythm and blood pressure.

# The Impact of Diet on Blood Pressure and Cholesterol

The intricate relationship between diet, blood pressure, and cholesterol is a central theme in the narrative of heart health. Understanding this relationship is crucial, as both high blood pressure (hypertension) and unbalanced cholesterol levels are silent harbors for cardiovascular diseases. Let's delve deeper into how dietary choices can significantly impact these critical health indicators.

## Managing Blood Pressure

High blood pressure, often termed the "silent killer," lacks obvious symptoms but can lead to severe heart conditions if left unmanaged. The role of diet in controlling blood pressure is substantial.

## Sodium and Blood Pressure

The excessive intake of sodium is a primary culprit in elevating blood pressure levels. Sodium, abundantly present in processed and fast foods, causes the body to retain water, thereby increasing the volume of blood and the pressure on arterial walls. This elevated pressure can strain the heart and damage blood vessels, increasing the risk of heart attack, stroke, and heart failure.

## DASH Diet and Blood Pressure

Conversely, diets such as the Dietary Approaches to Stop Hypertension (DASH) can significantly lower blood pressure. This diet emphasizes:

***Fruits and Vegetables:*** Rich in potassium, magnesium, and fiber, these foods help in managing blood pressure. Potassium, for example, lessens the effects of sodium and eases tension in blood vessel walls.

***Low-Fat Dairy:*** These products provide calcium and protein without the added risk of saturated fats.

Whole Grains: Being high in fiber, they help in maintaining a healthy blood pressure.

***Lean Protein:*** Sources like fish, poultry, and legumes are included, providing essential nutrients without unhealthy fats.

## Controlling Cholesterol

Cholesterol, a waxy substance found in your blood, is essential for building healthy cells. However, imbalances in cholesterol levels, particularly between Low-Density Lipoprotein (LDL, or "bad" cholesterol) and High-Density Lipoprotein (HDL, or "good" cholesterol), can lead to heart disease.

1.  **Saturated and Trans Fats**

Diets high in saturated and trans fats significantly contribute to the rise in LDL cholesterol. These fats are commonly found in:

*Fried Foods:* They often contain trans fats which increase LDL cholesterol.

*Baked Goods:* Many baked items are made with shortening or butter, high in saturated fats.

*Processed Snacks:* These can be high in both trans and saturated fats.

2.  **Diet Rich in Omega-3 Fatty Acids, Fiber, and Phytosterols**

To counteract the effects of bad cholesterol, incorporating foods rich in omega-3 fatty acids, fiber, and phytosterols is beneficial.

*Omega-3 Fatty Acids:* Found in fatty fish like salmon, mackerel, and in flaxseeds and walnuts, these fats help reduce triglycerides and lower the risk of heart rhythm abnormalities.

*Fiber:* Soluble fiber, found in foods like oats, beans, apples, and carrots, can reduce the absorption of cholesterol into the bloodstream.

*Phytosterols:* These compounds, found in plants, help block the absorption of cholesterol. They are present in vegetable oils, nuts, and seeds.

### 3. Lifestyle Considerations

Alongside diet, other lifestyle factors play a crucial role in managing blood pressure and cholesterol. Regular physical activity, maintaining a healthy weight, avoiding tobacco use, and limiting alcohol consumption are all essential components of heart health.

# CHAPTER 3

# IMPLEMENTING THE DASH DIET

## Foods to Embrace

### 1. Fruits and Vegetables:

- ***Servings and Variety:*** The recommendation of 4 to 5 servings of both fruits and vegetables daily underlines their importance in the DASH Diet. A serving could be a medium-sized apple, half a cup of cooked vegetables, or a cup of raw leafy greens. The variety is key; incorporating different colors and types ensures a wide range of nutrients.

- ***Benefits:*** These foods are high in essential vitamins, minerals, and fiber, while being low in calories. They help in maintaining a healthy blood pressure and reduce the risk of heart diseases.

### 2. Whole Grains:

- ***Servings and Choices:*** 6 to 8 servings of whole grains per day is recommended. One serving might be a slice of whole-wheat bread, half a cup of cooked brown rice or whole-grain pasta.

- ***Benefits:*** Whole grains are a good source of fiber and other nutrients that play a role in regulating blood pressure and heart health.

## 3. Dairy:

- ***Servings and Types:*** 2 to 3 servings of low-fat or fat-free dairy products are advised. This includes items like skim milk, low-fat yogurt, and low-fat cheese.

- ***Benefits:*** Dairy products provide calcium, vitamin D, and protein but choosing low-fat or fat-free options helps keep the saturated fat in check.

## 4. Lean Proteins:

- ***Servings and Sources:*** Limiting to 6 servings or less per day, lean proteins include skinless poultry, fish, and lean cuts of meat. Plant-based sources like tofu are also excellent choices.

- ***Benefits:*** These proteins provide essential amino acids without the high saturated fat content found in fattier cuts of meat.

## 5. Nuts, Seeds, and Legumes:

- *Frequency and Portions:* Recommended 4 to 5 times a week, nuts, seeds, and legumes are not just for snacking. They can be incorporated into meals in various ways.
- *Benefits:* These are rich in protein, fiber, magnesium, and other nutrients beneficial for heart health.

## 6. Fats and Oils:

- *Servings and Types:* With a recommendation of 2 to 3 servings a day, healthy oils like olive and canola oil are preferred. These should replace saturated fats found in butter and animal fat.
- *Benefits:* These oils provide essential fatty acids and help in the absorption of certain vitamins.

## Foods to Avoid or Limit

## 1. High Sodium Foods:

- *Examples:* This includes most processed foods like canned soups, frozen dinners, and deli meats, as well as fast food.

- ***Reasons to Avoid:*** High sodium intake is directly linked to high blood pressure, a risk factor for heart disease.

## 2. Sweets and Added Sugars:

- ***Examples:*** Limit sugary beverages, candies, cookies, and pastries.
- ***Reasons to Limit:*** These foods contribute to excess calorie intake and can lead to weight gain and elevated blood sugar levels, impacting heart health.

## 3. High-fat Dairy and Meats:

- ***Examples:*** Full-fat cheese, cream, and fatty cuts of meat like ribeye steak should be consumed less frequently.
- ***Reasons to Limit:*** These are high in saturated fats, which can raise cholesterol levels and increase the risk of heart disease.

## 4. Tropical Oils:

- ***Examples:*** Palm oil and coconut oil, though sometimes marketed as healthy, are high in saturated fats.

- ***Reasons to Use Sparingly:*** Despite their natural origin, these oils can contribute to elevated cholesterol levels.

## Implementing These Guidelines

Adopting the DASH Diet involves more than just knowing what foods to eat and avoid; it's about incorporating these guidelines into your daily life in a sustainable, enjoyable way. This means finding creative ways to increase fruits and vegetables in your diet, choosing whole grains over refined ones, and being mindful of the types of fats and proteins you consume. It also involves reading food labels to be aware of hidden sodium and sugars, even in foods that may seem healthy.

## Meal Planning Tips:

**Start Slow:** Gradually incorporate DASH-friendly foods into your diet. Start with adding one vegetable or fruit to each meal.

**Plan Your Meals:** Think ahead about what you'll eat during the week. Prepare DASH-friendly snacks like cut vegetables or a small handful of nuts.

**Watch Your Portions:** Use measuring cups or a kitchen scale to get used to the correct serving sizes.

**Cook at Home:** This gives you complete control over what goes into your food, especially the amount of salt.

**Be Creative:** Experiment with herbs and spices instead of salt to flavor your meals.

**Stay Hydrated:** Drink plenty of water. Limiting sugary drinks and alcohol is also part of the DASH Diet.

**Track Your Progress:** Keep a food diary to monitor your eating habits and make adjustments as needed.

# Breakfast Recipes for Heart Health

## 1. Spinach and Mushroom Omelette

**Ingredients:**

3 egg whites

1 cup fresh spinach, chopped

1/2 cup mushrooms, sliced

1 tbsp olive oil

Salt and pepper to taste

**Preparation Instructions:**

Heat olive oil in a non-stick skillet over medium heat.

Sauté mushrooms until tender.

Add spinach and cook until wilted.

In a bowl, whisk egg whites with salt and pepper.

Pour egg whites into the skillet, covering the spinach and mushrooms.

Cook until the eggs are set and fold the omelette in half.

Serve hot.

**Nutritional Information:**

Calories: 150

Protein: 14g

Fat: 9g

Sodium: 200mg

## 2. Berry Quinoa Breakfast Bowl

**Ingredients:**

1/2 cup cooked quinoa

1/2 cup mixed berries (blueberries, raspberries, strawberries)

1 tbsp chopped almonds

1/2 cup low-fat milk or almond milk

1 tsp honey (optional)

**Preparation Instructions:**

In a bowl, combine cooked quinoa with low-fat milk.

Top with mixed berries and chopped almonds.

Drizzle with honey for added sweetness if desired.

Serve immediately.

**Nutritional Information:**

Calories: 220

Protein: 8g

Fat: 5g

Sodium: 30mg

## 3. Avocado Toast on Whole Grain Bread

**Ingredients:**

2 slices whole grain bread

1 ripe avocado

1 tomato, sliced

Salt and pepper to taste

Red pepper flakes (optional)

**Preparation Instructions:**

Toast the whole grain bread to your liking.

Mash the avocado and spread evenly on the toasted bread.

Top with tomato slices.

Season with salt, pepper, and red pepper flakes if desired.

Serve immediately.

## Nutritional Information:

Calories: 250

Protein: 6g

Fat: 14g

Sodium: 180mg

## 4. Greek Yogurt with Honey and Walnuts

### Ingredients:

1 cup low-fat Greek yogurt

2 tbsp walnuts, chopped

1 tbsp honey

A pinch of cinnamon (optional)

### Preparation Instructions:

In a bowl, combine Greek yogurt with honey and a pinch of cinnamon.

Top with chopped walnuts.

Serve chilled.

**Nutritional Information:**

Calories: 200

Protein: 18g

Fat: 9g

Sodium: 60mg

**5. Veggie Breakfast Scramble**

**Ingredients:**

2 egg whites

1/2 cup bell peppers, diced

1/4 cup onions, diced

1/4 cup tomatoes, diced

1 tbsp olive oil

Salt and pepper to taste

**Preparation Instructions:**

In a skillet, heat olive oil over medium heat.

Sauté bell peppers and onions until tender.

Add tomatoes and cook for an additional minute.

Pour in egg whites, season with salt and pepper, and scramble.

Cook until the eggs are set.

Serve hot.

**Nutritional Information:**

Calories: 150

Protein: 10g

Fat: 9g

Sodium: 200mg

## 6. Banana Oatmeal Pancakes

**Ingredients:**

1 ripe banana, mashed

1/2 cup rolled oats

2 egg whites

1/2 tsp baking powder

1/4 tsp cinnamon

1/4 cup low-fat milk

**Preparation Instructions:**

In a blender, combine all ingredients and blend until smooth.

Heat a non-stick skillet over medium heat.

Pour batter to form pancakes and cook until bubbles form on top.

Flip and cook until golden brown.

Serve with fresh fruit or a drizzle of honey.

**Nutritional Information:**

Calories: 250

Protein: 10g

Fat: 4g

Sodium: 200mg

## 7. Chia Seed Pudding

**Ingredients:**

2 tbsp chia seeds

1/2 cup almond milk

1/2 tsp vanilla extract

1 tbsp honey

Fresh berries for topping

**Preparation Instructions:**

In a bowl, mix chia seeds, almond milk, vanilla extract, and honey.

Stir well and refrigerate overnight.

Top with fresh berries before serving.

**Nutritional Information:**

Calories: 200

Protein: 4g

Fat: 8g

Sodium: 30mg

## 8. Sweet Potato and Spinach Hash

**Ingredients:**

1 medium sweet potato, diced

1 cup spinach, chopped

1/2 onion, diced

1 clove garlic, minced

1 tbsp olive oil

Salt and pepper to taste

**Preparation Instructions:**

In a skillet, heat olive oil over medium heat.

Add sweet potato and onion, cook until tender.

Add garlic and spinach, cook until spinach is wilted.

Season with salt and pepper.

Serve hot.

**Nutritional Information:**

Calories: 180

Protein: 3g

Fat: 7g

Sodium: 70mg

# Lunch Recipes for Heart Health

## 1. Quinoa and Black Bean Salad

**Ingredients:**

1 cup quinoa

2 cups water

1 can black beans, drained and rinsed

1 red bell pepper, chopped

1/2 cup fresh cilantro, chopped

1/4 cup lime juice

2 tbsp olive oil

1 tsp cumin

Salt and pepper to taste

## Preparation Instructions:

Rinse quinoa under cold water. In a saucepan, bring water to a boil. Add quinoa, reduce heat to low, cover, and cook for 15 minutes.

In a large bowl, combine cooked quinoa, black beans, red bell pepper, and cilantro.

In a small bowl, whisk together lime juice, olive oil, cumin, salt, and pepper.

Pour dressing over quinoa mixture and toss to combine.

Serve chilled or at room temperature.

## Nutritional Information:

Calories: 220

Protein: 9g

Fat: 7g

Sodium: 150mg

## 2. Grilled Chicken and Vegetable Wrap

**Ingredients:**

2 boneless, skinless chicken breasts

1 zucchini, sliced

1 yellow squash, sliced

1 red onion, sliced

4 whole wheat tortillas

2 tbsp olive oil

1 tbsp balsamic vinegar

Salt and pepper to taste

**Preparation Instructions:**

Preheat grill to medium-high heat.

Brush chicken and vegetables with olive oil and balsamic vinegar. Season with salt and pepper.

Grill chicken for 6-7 minutes on each side or until cooked through. Grill vegetables until tender.

Slice chicken into strips. Divide chicken and vegetables among tortillas.

Roll up the wraps and serve.

**Nutritional Information:**

Calories: 350

Protein: 28g

Fat: 12g

Sodium: 200mg

**3. Mediterranean Chickpea Salad**

**Ingredients:**

1 can chickpeas, drained and rinsed

1 cucumber, diced

1/2 cup cherry tomatoes, halved

1/2 red onion, finely chopped

1/4 cup feta cheese, crumbled

1/4 cup parsley, chopped

3 tbsp olive oil

2 tbsp lemon juice

Salt and pepper to taste

**Preparation Instructions:**

In a large bowl, combine chickpeas, cucumber, cherry tomatoes, red onion, feta cheese, and parsley.

In a small bowl, whisk together olive oil and lemon juice. Season with salt and pepper.

Pour dressing over salad and toss to combine.

Serve chilled.

**Nutritional Information:**

Calories: 260

Protein: 9g

Fat: 14g

Sodium: 180mg

**4. Turkey and Avocado Sandwich**

**Ingredients:**

2 slices whole wheat bread

4 oz turkey breast, sliced

1/2 avocado, sliced

1 tomato, sliced

Lettuce leaves

1 tbsp mustard

Salt and pepper to taste

**Preparation Instructions:**

Toast the whole wheat bread slices.

Spread mustard on one slice of bread.

Layer turkey, avocado, tomato slices, and lettuce on the bread.

Top with the other slice of bread, cut in half, and serve.

**Nutritional Information:**

Calories: 330

Protein: 25g

Fat: 13g

Sodium: 250mg

**5. Lentil Soup with Spinach**

**Ingredients:**

1 cup dried lentils

4 cups vegetable broth

1 onion, chopped

2 garlic cloves, minced

2 carrots, diced

1 bunch of spinach, washed and chopped

2 tbsp olive oil

1 tsp ground cumin

Salt and pepper to taste

**Preparation Instructions:**

In a large pot, heat olive oil over medium heat. Add onion and garlic, sautéing until translucent.

Add carrots and cook for 5 minutes.

Stir in lentils, vegetable broth, cumin, salt, and pepper. Bring to a boil, then reduce heat and simmer for 20 minutes.

Add spinach and cook for an additional 5 minutes or until lentils are tender.

Serve hot.

**Nutritional Information:**

Calories: 230

Protein: 14g

Fat: 7g

Sodium: 300mg

## 6. Tuna and White Bean Salad

**Ingredients:**

2 cans of tuna in water, drained

1 can of white beans, drained and rinsed

1 red bell pepper, diced

2 celery stalks, diced

1/4 cup red onion, finely chopped

2 tbsp olive oil

1 tbsp lemon juice

1 tsp Dijon mustard

Salt and pepper to taste

Fresh parsley, chopped (for garnish)

**Preparation Instructions:**

In a large bowl, combine tuna, white beans, bell pepper, celery, and red onion.

In a small bowl, whisk together olive oil, lemon juice, and Dijon mustard. Season with salt and pepper.

Pour the dressing over the tuna mixture and gently toss to coat.

Garnish with fresh parsley before serving.

**Nutritional Information:**

Calories: 280

Protein: 25g

Fat: 10g

Sodium: 220mg

**7. Roasted Vegetable and Hummus Wrap**

**Ingredients:**

1 zucchini, sliced

1 red bell pepper, sliced

1 yellow bell pepper, sliced

1 eggplant, sliced

4 whole wheat tortillas

1 cup hummus

2 tbsp olive oil

Salt and pepper to taste

## Preparation Instructions:

Preheat oven to 400°F (200°C). Place sliced vegetables on a baking sheet, drizzle with olive oil, and season with salt and pepper.

Roast the vegetables for 20 minutes or until tender.

Spread each tortilla with a layer of hummus.

Divide the roasted vegetables among the tortillas, roll them up, and cut in half to serve.

## Nutritional Information:

Calories: 300

Protein: 10g

Fat: 15g

Sodium: 200mg

## 8. Spinach and Goat Cheese Stuffed Chicken

### Ingredients:

4 boneless, skinless chicken breasts

2 cups fresh spinach, chopped

1/2 cup goat cheese, crumbled

1 tbsp olive oil

1 tsp garlic powder

Salt and pepper to taste

**Preparation Instructions:**

Preheat oven to 375°F (190°C).

Make a pocket in each chicken breast by cutting along the side.

Mix spinach and goat cheese, and stuff into the chicken pockets. Secure with toothpicks.

Rub chicken with olive oil, garlic powder, salt, and pepper.

Bake for 25-30 minutes or until chicken is cooked through.

**Nutritional Information:**

Calories: 320

Protein: 35g

Fat: 17g

Sodium: 200mg

**9. Sweet Potato and Black Bean Burrito Bowl**

**Ingredients:** 2 sweet potatoes, peeled and cubed

1 can black beans, drained and rinsed

1 cup brown rice, cooked

1 avocado, sliced

1/2 cup corn kernels

1 lime, juiced

2 tbsp olive oil

1 tsp chili powder

Salt and pepper to taste

Fresh cilantro, chopped (for garnish)

## Preparation Instructions:

Preheat oven to 400°F (200°C). Toss sweet potatoes with 1 tbsp olive oil, chili powder, salt, and pepper. Roast for 25 minutes or until tender.

In a bowl, layer cooked brown rice, black beans, roasted sweet potatoes, corn, and avocado slices.

Drizzle with remaining olive oil and lime juice.

Garnish with fresh cilantro before serving.

## Nutritional Information:

Calories: 350

Protein: 10g

Fat: 12g

Sodium: 250mg

# Dinner Recipes for Heart Health

## Grilled Chicken and Quinoa Salad

## Ingredients:

4 skinless, boneless chicken breasts

1 cup quinoa

2 cups mixed salad greens

1 cucumber, sliced

1 red bell pepper, diced

2 tbsp balsamic vinegar

1 tbsp olive oil

Salt and pepper to taste

## Preparation Instructions:

Cook quinoa as per package instructions and let it cool.

Grill chicken breasts over medium heat until cooked through.

In a large bowl, combine quinoa, salad greens, cucumber, and red bell pepper.

Slice grilled chicken and add to the salad.

Drizzle with olive oil and balsamic vinegar.

Season with salt and pepper to taste.

**Nutritional Information:**

Calories: 350

Protein: 30g

Fat: 10g

Sodium: 150mg

**Lentil and Vegetable Stew**

**Ingredients:**

1 cup dry lentils

1 onion, chopped

2 carrots, diced

2 celery stalks, diced

1 can diced tomatoes (no salt added)

3 cups vegetable broth (low sodium)

1 tsp thyme

1 tsp rosemary

Salt and pepper to taste

**Preparation Instructions:**

Rinse lentils and set aside.

In a large pot, sauté onion, carrots, and celery until soft.

Add lentils, diced tomatoes, and vegetable broth.

Bring to a boil, then reduce heat and simmer for about 30 minutes.

Add thyme, rosemary, salt, and pepper.

Cook until lentils are tender.

**Nutritional Information:**

Calories: 220

Protein: 15g

Fat: 2g

Sodium: 200mg

**Turmeric Cauliflower and Chickpea Curry**

**Ingredients:** 1 head cauliflower, cut into florets

1 can chickpeas, drained and rinsed

1 onion, diced

2 cloves garlic, minced

1 can coconut milk (light)

2 tsp turmeric

1 tsp cumin

1 tsp coriander

Salt and pepper to taste

2 cups spinach

**Preparation Instructions:**

In a large skillet, sauté onion and garlic until translucent.

Add turmeric, cumin, and coriander, cook for 1 minute.

Add cauliflower, chickpeas, and coconut milk. Bring to a simmer.

Cook for 15 minutes or until cauliflower is tender.

Stir in spinach until wilted.

Season with salt and pepper.

**Nutritional Information:**

Calories: 260

Protein: 12g

Fat: 8g

Sodium: 150mg

## Stuffed Bell Peppers with Brown Rice and Vegetables

### Ingredients:

4 bell peppers, tops cut off and seeds removed

1 cup brown rice, cooked

1 zucchini, diced

1 cup black beans, cooked

1 cup corn kernels

1 tsp paprika

Salt and pepper to taste

1/2 cup shredded low-fat cheese

### Preparation Instructions:

Preheat oven to 375°F (190°C).

In a bowl, mix cooked brown rice, zucchini, black beans, corn, and paprika.

Stuff each bell pepper with the rice mixture.

Place stuffed peppers in a baking dish and cover with foil.

Bake for 30 minutes.

Remove foil, top each pepper with cheese, and bake for another 10 minutes.

## Nutritional Information:

Calories: 280

Protein: 15g

Fat: 5g

Sodium: 200mg

## Baked Cod with Tomato and Olive Tapenade

### Ingredients:

4 cod fillets (6 oz each)

1 cup cherry tomatoes, halved

1/4 cup olives, chopped

2 tbsp capers

1 tbsp olive oil

Salt and pepper to taste

### Preparation Instructions:

Preheat oven to 400°F (200°C).

Place cod fillets in a baking dish.

In a bowl, mix tomatoes, olives, capers, and olive oil.

Spoon the tapenade over the cod fillets.

Season with salt and pepper.

Bake for 15-20 minutes or until cod is cooked through.

**Nutritional Information:**

Calories: 220

Protein: 30g

Fat: 8g

Sodium: 300mg

**Vegetable Stir-Fry with Tofu and Brown Rice**

**Ingredients:** 1 block firm tofu, cubed

2 cups brown rice, cooked

1 red bell pepper, sliced

1 cup broccoli florets

1 carrot, sliced

2 tbsp low-sodium soy sauce

1 tbsp sesame oil

1 tsp ginger, grated

1 clove garlic, minced

**Preparation Instructions:**

In a large pan, heat sesame oil over medium heat.

Add tofu and cook until golden brown. Remove and set aside.

In the same pan, add garlic, ginger, and vegetables. Stir-fry until vegetables are tender.

Add cooked tofu, brown rice, and soy sauce to the pan. Stir well to combine.

Cook for an additional 5 minutes.

**Nutritional Information:**

Calories: 300

Protein: 18g

Fat: 10g

Sodium: 200mg

**Spinach and Mushroom Frittata**

**Ingredients:** 4 eggs

1 cup fresh spinach, chopped

1 cup mushrooms, sliced

1/4 cup low-fat milk

1/4 cup shredded low-fat cheese

1 tbsp olive oil

Salt and pepper to taste

**Preparation Instructions:**

Preheat oven to 350°F (175°C).

In a skillet, heat olive oil over medium heat. Add mushrooms and cook until tender.

Add spinach and cook until wilted.

In a bowl, whisk together eggs, milk, salt, and pepper.

Pour the egg mixture over the vegetables in the skillet.

Sprinkle cheese on top.

Transfer skillet to the oven and bake for 20 minutes or until the eggs are set.

**Nutritional Information:**

Calories: 200

Protein: 16g

Fat: 12g

Sodium: 220mg

# Snacks Recipes for Heart Health

## 1. Avocado and Tomato Salsa

**Ingredients:**

1 ripe avocado, diced

2 medium tomatoes, diced

1/4 cup red onion, finely chopped

1/4 cup cilantro, chopped

Juice of 1 lime

Salt and pepper to taste

**Preparation Instructions:**

In a bowl, combine avocado, tomatoes, red onion, and cilantro.

Squeeze lime juice over the mixture and stir gently.

Season with salt and pepper.

Serve with whole-grain tortilla chips or sliced vegetables.

**Nutritional Information:**

Calories: 50 per serving

Protein: 1g

Fat: 4g

Sodium: 5mg

## 2. Greek Yogurt with Mixed Berries

**Ingredients:** 1 cup low-fat Greek yogurt

1/2 cup mixed berries (strawberries, blueberries, raspberries)

1 tbsp honey (optional)

**Preparation Instructions:** Spoon Greek yogurt into a bowl.

Top with mixed berries.

Drizzle honey over the top if desired.

**Nutritional Information:**

Calories: 150

Protein: 12g

Fat: 1g

## 3. Almond and Date Energy Balls

**Ingredients:** 1 cup almonds

1 cup dates, pitted

1/4 cup unsweetened cocoa powder

1 tsp vanilla extract

**Preparation Instructions:** In a food processor, blend almonds and dates until they form a sticky mixture.

Add cocoa powder and vanilla extract, and blend until well combined.

Roll the mixture into small balls.

Refrigerate for at least 1 hour before serving.

**Nutritional Information:**

Calories: 90 per ball

Protein: 2g

Fat: 5g

**4. Carrot and Hummus Dip**

**Ingredients:**

2 cups baby carrots

1 cup hummus

**Preparation Instructions:**

Serve baby carrots with a side of hummus for dipping.

**Nutritional Information:**

Calories: 100 (for 10 carrots and 2 tbsp hummus)

Protein: 3g

Fat: 6g

## 5. Whole Grain Toast with Avocado

**Ingredients:**

1 slice whole-grain bread, toasted

1/2 avocado, mashed

Salt and pepper to taste

**Preparation Instructions:**

Spread mashed avocado on toasted bread.

Season with salt and pepper.

**Nutritional Information:**

Calories: 200

Protein: 6g

Fat: 10g

Sodium: 150mg

## 6. Cottage Cheese and Pineapple

**Ingredients:**

1/2 cup low-fat cottage cheese

1/2 cup pineapple chunks

**Preparation Instructions:**

Mix cottage cheese with pineapple chunks.

**Nutritional Information:**

Calories: 120

Protein: 12g

Fat: 1g

Sodium: 200mg

## 7. Baked Kale Chips

**Ingredients:**

1 bunch kale, washed and torn into bite-sized pieces

1 tbsp olive oil

Salt to taste

**Preparation Instructions:**

Preheat oven to 350°F (175°C).

Toss kale with olive oil and salt.

Spread on a baking sheet and bake for 10-15 minutes, until edges are crisp.

**Nutritional Information:**

Calories: 50 per serving

Protein: 2g

Fat: 3g

Sodium: 50mg

## 8. Whole Grain Rice Cakes with Peanut Butter

**Ingredients:**

2 whole grain rice cakes

2 tbsp natural peanut butter

**Preparation Instructions:**

Spread peanut butter evenly on rice cakes.

**Nutritional Information:**

Calories: 180

Protein: 8g

Fat: 10g

## 9. Roasted Chickpeas

**Ingredients:**

1 can chickpeas, drained and rinsed

1 tbsp olive oil

1/2 tsp paprika

Salt to taste

**Preparation Instructions:** Preheat oven to 400°F (200°C).

Toss chickpeas with olive oil, paprika, and salt.

Spread on a baking sheet and roast for 20-30 minutes until crispy.

**Nutritional Information:**

Calories: 120 per 1/4 cup serving

Protein: 6g

Fat: 4g

Sodium: 200mg

## 10. Sliced Bell Peppers with Guacamole

**Ingredients:** 1 bell pepper, sliced

1/2 cup guacamole

**Preparation Instructions:**

Serve sliced bell peppers with guacamole for dipping.

**Nutritional Information:**

Calories: 100 (for 1/2 pepper and 2 tbsp guacamole)

Protein: 2g

Fat: 8g

Sodium: 60mg

## 21 Days DASH Diet Meal Plan for Heart Health

**Day 1:**

- Breakfast: Greek Yogurt with Mixed Berries
- Lunch: Baked Salmon with Asparagus
- Dinner: Whole Grain Toast with Avocado
- Snacks: Avocado and Tomato Salsa, Almond and Date Energy Balls

**Day 2:**

- Breakfast: Whole Grain Toast with Avocado
- Lunch: Cottage Cheese and Pineapple
- Dinner: Baked Salmon with Asparagus

- Snacks: Carrot and Hummus Dip, Greek Yogurt with Mixed Berries

**Day 3:**

- Breakfast: Greek Yogurt with Mixed Berries
- Lunch: Whole Grain Rice Cakes with Peanut Butter
- Dinner: Baked Salmon with Asparagus
- Snacks: Sliced Bell Peppers with Guacamole, Almond and Date Energy Balls

**Day 4:**

- Breakfast: Whole Grain Toast with Avocado
- Lunch: Baked Salmon with Asparagus
- Dinner: Cottage Cheese and Pineapple
- Snacks: Greek Yogurt with Mixed Berries, Carrot and Hummus Dip

**Day 5:**

- Breakfast: Greek Yogurt with Mixed Berries
- Lunch: Cottage Cheese and Pineapple
- Dinner: Whole Grain Rice Cakes with Peanut Butter
- Snacks: Avocado and Tomato Salsa, Baked Kale Chips

**Day 6:**

- Breakfast: Whole Grain Toast with Avocado
- Lunch: Baked Salmon with Asparagus
- Dinner: Whole Grain Rice Cakes with Peanut Butter
- Snacks: Almond and Date Energy Balls, Sliced Bell Peppers with Guacamole

**Day 7:**

- Breakfast: Greek Yogurt with Mixed Berries
- Lunch: Cottage Cheese and Pineapple
- Dinner: Baked Salmon with Asparagus
- Snacks: Roasted Chickpeas, Carrot and Hummus Dip

**Day 8:**

- Breakfast: Whole Grain Toast with Avocado
- Lunch: Baked Salmon with Asparagus
- Dinner: Cottage Cheese and Pineapple
- Snacks: Greek Yogurt with Mixed Berries, Baked Kale Chips

**Day 9:**

- Breakfast: Greek Yogurt with Mixed Berries

- Lunch: Whole Grain Rice Cakes with Peanut Butter
- Dinner: Baked Salmon with Asparagus
- Snacks: Avocado and Tomato Salsa, Almond and Date Energy Balls

**Day 10:**

- Breakfast: Whole Grain Toast with Avocado
- Lunch: Cottage Cheese and Pineapple
- Dinner: Whole Grain Rice Cakes with Peanut Butter
- Snacks: Sliced Bell Peppers with Guacamole, Carrot and Hummus Dip

**Day 11:**

- Breakfast: Greek Yogurt with Mixed Berries
- Lunch: Baked Salmon with Asparagus
- Dinner: Whole Grain Toast with Avocado
- Snacks: Roasted Chickpeas, Almond and Date Energy Balls

**Day 12:**

- Breakfast: Whole Grain Toast with Avocado
- Lunch: Cottage Cheese and Pineapple
- Dinner: Baked Salmon with Asparagus

- Snacks: Greek Yogurt with Mixed Berries, Baked Kale Chips

**Day 13:**

- Breakfast: Greek Yogurt with Mixed Berries
- Lunch: Whole Grain Rice Cakes with Peanut Butter
- Dinner: Cottage Cheese and Pineapple
- Snacks: Avocado and Tomato Salsa, Carrot and Hummus Dip

**Day 14:**

- Breakfast: Whole Grain Toast with Avocado
- Lunch: Baked Salmon with Asparagus
- Dinner: Whole Grain Rice Cakes with Peanut Butter
- Snacks: Sliced Bell Peppers with Guacamole, Almond and Date Energy Balls

**Day 15:**

- Breakfast: Greek Yogurt with Mixed Berries
- Lunch: Cottage Cheese and Pineapple
- Dinner: Baked Salmon with Asparagus
- Snacks: Roasted Chickpeas, Baked Kale Chips

**Day 16:**

- Breakfast: Whole Grain Toast with Avocado
- Lunch: Whole Grain Rice Cakes with Peanut Butter
- Dinner: Cottage Cheese and Pineapple
- Snacks: Greek Yogurt with Mixed Berries, Avocado and Tomato Salsa

**Day 17:**

- Breakfast: Greek Yogurt with Mixed Berries
- Lunch: Baked Salmon with Asparagus
- Dinner: Whole Grain Toast with Avocado
- Snacks: Carrot and Hummus Dip, Almond and Date Energy Balls

**Day 18:**

- Breakfast: Whole Grain Toast with Avocado
- Lunch: Cottage Cheese and Pineapple
- Dinner: Baked Salmon with Asparagus
- Snacks: Sliced Bell Peppers with Guacamole, Greek Yogurt with Mixed Berries

**Day 19:**

- Breakfast: Greek Yogurt with Mixed Berries

- Lunch: Whole Grain Rice Cakes with Peanut Butter
- Dinner: Cottage Cheese and Pineapple
- Snacks: Avocado and Tomato Salsa, Roasted Chickpeas

**Day 20:**

- Breakfast: Whole Grain Toast with Avocado
- Lunch: Baked Salmon with Asparagus
- Dinner: Whole Grain Rice Cakes with Peanut Butter
- Snacks: Almond and Date Energy Balls, Baked Kale Chips

**Day 21:**

- Breakfast: Greek Yogurt with Mixed Berries
- Lunch: Cottage Cheese and Pineapple
- Dinner: Baked Salmon with Asparagus
- Snacks: Carrot and Hummus Dip, Sliced Bell Peppers with Guacamole

# CHAPTER 4

# ADAPTING THE DASH DIET TO YOUR LIFESTYLE

## Practical Tips for Grocery Shopping

### 1. Plan Ahead

a) **Meal Planning:** Before your grocery trip, sit down and plan your meals for the week. This includes all meals and snacks. Utilize DASH-friendly recipes and consider your schedule; on busier days, plan simpler meals or leftovers.

b) **Make a List:** Based on your meal plan, create a detailed shopping list. This helps you stay focused and resist the temptation of unhealthy impulse purchases.

c) **Check Pantry First:** Before finalizing your list, check your pantry and refrigerator to avoid buying what you already have. This also helps in reducing food waste.

### 2. Stick to the Perimeter

a) **Fresh Produce:** Start your shopping trip in the produce section. Load up on a variety of fruits and vegetables, as they are cornerstones of the DASH Diet. Aim for color and variety to ensure a range of nutrients.

b) **Dairy and Meats:** After produce, move to the dairy and meat sections. Choose lean meats and low-fat dairy options. Remember, the goal is to reduce saturated fat intake.

c) **Avoid Processed Foods:** By shopping the perimeter, you naturally avoid many processed foods high in sodium and unhealthy fats, typically found in the center aisles.

## 3. Read Labels

a) **Understand Nutrition Labels:** Learn to read and understand nutrition labels. Look at the sodium content, keeping in mind the daily limit recommended by the DASH Diet.

b) **Check for Additives:** Apart from sodium, check for added sugars and unhealthy fats like trans fats. These can negate the heart-healthy benefits of your diet.

c) **Ingredients List:** The fewer the ingredients, and the more recognizable they are, the better.

## 4. Buy Fresh or Frozen Vegetables

a) **Seasonal Choices:** Opt for seasonal produce as they tend to be fresher and more affordable.

b) **Frozen Options:** When fresh isn't available or practical, choose frozen vegetables without added salt or sauces. They are a great alternative and can be just as nutritious.

## 5. Choose Whole Grains

a) **Identify Whole Grains:** Look for products where the first ingredient listed is a whole grain. Be wary of labels that say "made with whole grains" as they may only contain small amounts.

b) **Diverse Options:** Explore different whole grains like quinoa, barley, and bulgur. They offer variety and can be used in multiple recipes.

## 6. Select Lean Proteins

a) **Variety in Protein:** Balance your protein intake by including both animal and plant sources. Plant-based proteins also add fiber, which is beneficial for heart health.

b) **Fish Choices:** When selecting fish, consider fatty fish like salmon, which are high in heart-healthy omega-3 fatty acids.

## 7. Don't Forget Dairy

a) **Calcium-Rich Foods:** Apart from milk, look for other calcium-rich foods like yogurt and cheese, opting for low-fat versions.

b) **Alternative Dairy Products:** If you're lactose intolerant or vegan, explore calcium-fortified alternatives like almond or soy milk.

## 8. Use Herbs and Spices

a) **Flavorful Additions:** Herbs and spices can add immense flavor without the need for salt. Experiment with different combinations to find what you like.

b) **Salt Substitutes:** Be cautious with salt substitutes, especially if you have kidney problems or are on certain medications. Always consult with a healthcare provider.

# Cooking and Meal Prep for the DASH Diet

## 1. Embrace Home Cooking

Cooking at home is at the heart of the DASH Diet. It allows for full control over what goes into your food, ensuring adherence to low sodium and low saturated fat guidelines. Start by setting up your kitchen with DASH-friendly ingredients like fresh vegetables, fruits, whole grains, lean meats, and low-fat dairy products. Invest in a good set of non-stick cookware and a variety of spices to make your cooking experiences both enjoyable and healthy. Plan your meals around the DASH Diet's emphasis on vegetables and whole grains, and experiment with different cooking techniques like grilling, baking, or steaming to keep your meals interesting and diverse.

## 2. Batch Cooking

Batch cooking is incredibly effective for maintaining a consistent DASH Diet. Dedicate a day of the week to prepare large quantities of DASH-friendly meals. Cook a big pot of brown rice or quinoa, roast a variety of vegetables, grill chicken breasts, and prepare a week's worth of salad greens. Store these in portion-controlled containers. This approach not only saves time during the week but also helps resist the temptation of less healthy, convenience food options.

## 3. Slow Cooking and One-Pot Meals

Slow cookers and one-pot meals are a boon for anyone on the DASH Diet. These cooking methods allow for the natural flavors of foods to develop, reducing the need for added salt and fat. Try making a hearty stew with lean meats and a variety of vegetables, or a vegetarian chili with beans and legumes. These methods also allow for the easy incorporation of a variety of spices and herbs, adding depth and complexity to your meals without compromising health.

## 4. Experiment with New Recipes

The DASH Diet is an opportunity to explore culinary diversity. Look for recipes from different cultures that focus on fresh ingredients and robust flavors. For instance, Mediterranean cuisine, with its emphasis on vegetables, fish, and olive oil, aligns well with the DASH Diet. Asian recipes can be adapted by reducing sodium and increasing vegetables and lean proteins. Be adventurous with herbs and spices; they are a healthy way to add flavor without adding salt or fat.

## 5. Portion Control

Even on the DASH Diet, it's important to be mindful of portion sizes. Use measuring cups, scales, or visual cues (like the size of your palm or fist) to ensure appropriate serving sizes. Remember that vegetables should make up the largest portion of your plate, followed by whole grains and lean protein. By controlling portion sizes, you can enjoy a variety of foods without overeating.

## 6. Healthy Substitutions

Making healthy substitutions is a key strategy in the DASH Diet. Replace high-fat ingredients with healthier alternatives without sacrificing flavor. For instance, use Greek yogurt in place of sour cream for a creamy, tangy flavor with less fat and more protein. Mashed avocado can replace butter in some recipes, providing healthy fats and a creamy texture. Other substitutions include using whole wheat flour instead of white flour, applesauce or mashed bananas for some of the oil or butter in baked goods, and herbs or lemon juice in place of salt.

# DASH Diet for Different Age Groups and Health Conditions

## 1. Children and Adolescents

Introducing the DASH Diet early in life sets a foundation for healthy eating habits that can last a lifetime. For children and adolescents, the focus should be on integrating a wide range of fruits, vegetables, and whole grains into their daily meals. This not only ensures they get a variety of essential nutrients but also helps in developing their taste preferences for healthier food choices.

### *Practical Approaches:*

- **Make Nutrition Fun:** Use colorful fruits and vegetables to create visually appealing meals. Engaging children in choosing produce can make them more interested in eating healthily.

- **Educational Cooking:** Involve children in meal preparation. Simple tasks like washing vegetables or mixing ingredients can be educational and fun.

- **Balanced Snacking:** Offer healthy snacks like carrot sticks, apple slices, or whole-grain crackers to maintain energy levels between meals.

## 2. Adults and Seniors

For adults, the DASH Diet is an effective tool for managing or preventing hypertension and other cardiovascular diseases. As adults age into their senior years, their nutritional needs evolve. Seniors may require higher intakes of calcium and vitamin D for bone health, which the DASH Diet can support.

*Adaptations for Seniors:*

- **Easy-to-Chew Options:** Soft-cooked vegetables and tender meats can be more manageable for seniors with dental issues.

- **Nutrient-Dense Foods:** Foods high in fiber, protein, and essential nutrients, but low in calories, are ideal for seniors who may have lower energy needs.

- **Hydration Focus:** Ensuring adequate fluid intake is crucial for seniors, particularly when increasing fiber intake.

## 3. Pregnant and Nursing Women

The nutrient-rich nature of the DASH Diet makes it beneficial for pregnant and nursing women. However, they should consult their healthcare providers for personalized advice, as their nutritional requirements are higher.

***Special Considerations:***

- **Increased Caloric Needs:** Pregnant and nursing women may need more calories. Incorporating nutrient-dense, higher-calorie foods like nuts, seeds, and avocados can help meet these needs.

- **Focus on Key Nutrients:** Folate, iron, calcium, and omega-3 fatty acids are crucial during pregnancy and breastfeeding. Emphasizing foods rich in these nutrients is important.

## 4. Individuals with Chronic Health Conditions

For those with chronic conditions such as diabetes, kidney disease, or food allergies, the DASH Diet can often be customized to align with their specific dietary needs.

**Customization Strategies:**

- **Diabetes Management:** The DASH Diet's emphasis on whole grains and fiber-rich foods can aid in blood sugar control. Monitoring carbohydrate intake and ensuring balanced meals can be particularly beneficial.

- **Kidney Disease Considerations:** Depending on the stage of kidney disease, adjustments in potassium and protein intake might be necessary. Consulting with a dietitian is crucial.

- **Allergy Adaptations:** For those with food allergies, alternative sources of nutrients found in the allergenic foods can be identified and incorporated into the diet.

# CHAPTER 5

# TRACKING YOUR PROGRESS

## Setting Realistic Goals

The foundation of any successful health journey lies in setting achievable and meaningful goals. Realistic goals provide direction and motivation, helping you stay focused and committed to your dietary changes.

- **Start with Clear, Achievable Objectives:** Goals should be specific and attainable. Instead of setting a vague goal like "I want to be healthier," aim for something more tangible, such as "I want to reduce my blood pressure by 10 points in the next three months."

- **Make Your Goals Measurable:** Incorporate ways to measure your progress. For instance, if your goal is to incorporate more vegetables into your diet, you might set a target of including at least three different vegetables in your meals each day.

- **Be Patient and Realistic:** Understand that changes, especially those related to health and diet, take time. Setting overly ambitious or unrealistic goals can lead to disappointment and demotivation.

- **Customize Your Goals:** Your goals should align with your personal health needs and lifestyle. If you are a busy professional, preparing complex meals every day might not be feasible, so your goal could be to prepare a week's worth of DASH-friendly meals during the weekend.

- **Review and Adjust Your Goals Regularly:** As you progress, your needs and abilities might change. Regularly revisiting and adjusting your goals ensures they remain relevant and challenging.

## Monitoring Blood Pressure and Cholesterol Levels

Two critical health indicators that you should monitor while on the DASH Diet are blood pressure and cholesterol levels. These metrics provide direct feedback on the impact of your dietary changes on your heart health.

- **Regular Blood Pressure Monitoring:** High blood pressure, or hypertension, is a silent health issue that often goes unnoticed. Regular monitoring, either at home with a blood pressure monitor or through visits to your healthcare provider, is essential. Keeping a log of your readings can help you and your healthcare provider see the effects of dietary changes over time.

- **Understanding Cholesterol Levels:** Cholesterol levels, particularly LDL (bad cholesterol) and HDL (good cholesterol), are crucial indicators of heart health. Regular blood tests, as recommended by your healthcare provider, are necessary to monitor these levels.

- **Interpreting the Numbers:** Understanding what your blood pressure and cholesterol levels mean is crucial. For blood pressure, readings below 120/80 mm Hg are considered normal, while for cholesterol, LDL levels should be low, and HDL levels should be high.

- **Correlating Diet and Health Metrics:** Keep a food diary alongside your health metrics log. This practice helps in understanding how specific dietary changes are affecting your blood pressure and cholesterol levels.

## Adjusting the Diet as Needed

### Listening to Your Body

The principle of listening to your body is pivotal in making the DASH Diet work for you. Every individual's body reacts differently to various foods and portions. For instance:

- **Identifying Food Sensitivities:** Some might find that dairy products, despite being a part of the DASH Diet, cause discomfort or bloating. In such cases, it's advisable to try lactose-free options or plant-based alternatives.

- **Noticing Energy Levels:** Paying attention to how different foods affect your energy levels throughout the day can be insightful. If a certain food leaves you feeling sluggish, it might be worth reducing its intake.

- **Gastrointestinal Reactions:** Foods that cause gastrointestinal distress, such as excessive gas or constipation, should be consumed in moderation or replaced with more suitable alternatives.

## Balancing Macronutrients

The DASH Diet focuses on a balanced intake of macronutrients – carbohydrates, proteins, and fats – but individual needs can vary greatly:

- **Carbohydrates:** While whole grains are a staple in the DASH Diet, some individuals may need to adjust their carbohydrate intake, particularly if managing conditions like diabetes or aiming for weight loss.

- **Proteins:** The type and amount of protein can be adjusted based on personal health goals, activity levels, and dietary preferences. For instance, vegetarians might rely on legumes and soy products instead of meat.

- **Fats:** The DASH Diet recommends healthy fats, but the quantity might need tweaking depending on factors like cholesterol levels or specific dietary goals.

## Incorporating Variety

A diverse diet is not only nutritionally beneficial but also helps in maintaining interest and adherence to the diet:

- **Trying New Foods:** Regularly incorporating different fruits, vegetables, and whole grains can prevent dietary boredom. Experimenting with seasonal produce can add excitement to meals.

- **Creative Cooking:** Exploring various cuisines and cooking techniques can introduce new flavors and textures, making the dietary experience enjoyable and diverse.

## Seeking Professional Advice

Consulting a healthcare professional or dietician is particularly important in certain situations:

- **Health Conditions:** Those with specific health issues, such as kidney disease, diabetes, or food allergies, should seek advice to ensure the diet aligns with their health requirements.

- **Customization for Goals:** A dietician can provide tailored advice for those with specific objectives like weight loss, muscle gain, or improved athletic performance.

## Adjusting for Lifestyle Changes

Life changes often bring about shifts in nutritional needs and opportunities for dietary adjustments:

- **New Job or Schedule:** A change in work schedule might affect meal times and energy requirements. Adapting meal planning and preparation to fit the new routine is crucial.

- **Stress and Emotional Well-Being:** Stress can impact dietary choices and appetite. Recognizing these changes and adjusting the diet accordingly can help in managing stress better.

- **Age-Related Adjustments:** As you age, your nutritional needs, appetite, and digestion might change. The diet may need adjustments in terms of fiber intake, calorie needs, and nutrient density.

- **Physical Activity Levels:** Increased physical activity necessitates higher energy and protein intake. Conversely, a more sedentary lifestyle might call for a reduction in overall caloric intake.

# Part II
# Beyond diet

# CHAPTER 6

# COMPLEMENTARY LIFESTYLE CHANGES

## Exercise and the DASH Diet

The interplay between exercise and nutrition is a cornerstone of maintaining and improving heart health. While the DASH Diet provides a comprehensive guide on what to eat, integrating exercise into this dietary plan is crucial for optimal results. Exercise not only complements the nutritional aspect of the DASH Diet but also enhances the body's ability to utilize the nutrients consumed. Here, we delve deeper into how exercise synergizes with the DASH Diet and the types of exercise that are most beneficial.

### The Synergy of Exercise and Nutrition

Exercise and nutrition are two sides of the same coin when it comes to heart health. The DASH Diet, with its focus on nutrient-rich foods, lays the foundation for a healthy heart by regulating the intake of essential nutrients. However, it is through exercise that these nutrients are optimally utilized. Regular physical activity improves cardiovascular efficiency, boosts metabolism, and aids in weight management, enhancing the benefits of a heart-healthy diet.

**Cardiovascular Health:** Exercise strengthens the heart muscle, improves blood circulation, and helps in reducing blood pressure and cholesterol levels. When combined with the DASH Diet's emphasis on low-sodium and nutrient-dense foods, the result is a significantly lower risk of heart disease.

**Metabolism Enhancement:** Physical activity increases the body's metabolic rate, meaning it burns calories more efficiently. This is particularly important in utilizing the energy provided by the healthy carbohydrates and fats recommended in the DASH Diet.

**Weight Management:** Maintaining a healthy weight is crucial for heart health. Exercise, in combination with the DASH Diet, helps in achieving and sustaining a healthy weight, thereby reducing the strain on the heart.

**Types of Beneficial Exercise**

Different forms of exercise contribute to heart health in various ways, and incorporating a mix of these can offer comprehensive benefits:

- **Aerobic Exercises:** Activities like brisk walking, jogging, swimming, or cycling are stellar for cardiovascular health. They increase the heart rate, improving the heart's pumping efficiency and endurance. Aerobic exercises also play a significant role in burning calories and managing weight, which is vital for reducing the strain on the heart.

- **Strength Training:** Incorporating strength training, such as using weights or resistance bands, at least two days a week, is essential for building and maintaining lean muscle mass. Muscle tissue burns more calories than fat tissue, even at rest, thus boosting overall metabolism. This type of exercise also helps in managing blood sugar levels, a key factor in overall heart health, especially for those with or at risk of diabetes.

- **Flexibility and Balance Exercises:** Practices like yoga and stretching are not just about flexibility; they also contribute to heart health. They help in reducing muscle tension, improving posture, and enhancing joint mobility. This type of exercise is also beneficial for stress reduction, which is crucial for a healthy heart.

## Creating a Sustainable Routine

The key to reaping the benefits of exercise in conjunction with the DASH Diet is consistency and sustainability. It's not about engaging in intense, exhaustive workouts but rather about integrating physical activity into your daily routine in a way that is enjoyable and sustainable.

**Finding Enjoyable Activities:** The best exercise is the one you enjoy and will stick with. Whether it's a dance class, a nightly walk, or a weekend bike ride, the goal is to find activities that you look forward to.

**Setting Realistic Goals:** Start with achievable goals. If you're new to exercise, begin with shorter sessions and gradually increase the duration and intensity.

**Mixing It Up:** Incorporate different types of exercises to keep your routine interesting and to work on different aspects of fitness.

**Accountability:** Having a workout partner or joining a group can increase your motivation and commitment to regular exercise.

**Listen to Your Body:** It's important to pay attention to your body's signals. Rest when you need to and avoid pushing yourself too hard, especially if you're just starting out.

## Stress Management Techniques

In the fast-paced world we live in, stress is an inevitable part of life. However, its impact on our health, particularly heart health, can be profound and far-reaching. Chronic stress, a persistent state of mental or emotional strain, is particularly harmful. It can lead to high blood pressure, a major contributor to heart disease. Additionally, stress often drives individuals towards unhealthy coping mechanisms like overeating or indulging in unhealthy foods, behaviors that can directly counteract the benefits of heart-healthy diets such as the DASH Diet.

### Understanding the Impact of Stress

The connection between stress and heart health is complex yet significant. Under stress, the body produces higher levels of cortisol and adrenaline, hormones that increase heart rate and blood pressure, preparing the body for a 'fight or flight' response. While this response can be beneficial in short bursts, prolonged stress means these hormones are continually elevated, leading to chronic high blood pressure and straining the heart and arteries.

Moreover, stress influences behaviors and lifestyle choices. Many people under stress may turn to high-calorie, high-sodium, and high-fat comfort foods – precisely the types of foods the DASH Diet aims to limit. This dietary shift can undo the benefits of the DASH Diet, increasing the risk of heart disease.

**Techniques to Manage Stress**

Managing stress is a multifaceted approach, involving both psychological and physical strategies:

- **Mindfulness and Meditation:** These practices are powerful tools for centering the mind, reducing anxiety, and improving emotional regulation. Mindfulness involves being fully present in the moment, aware of where we are and what we're doing, without being overly reactive or overwhelmed by what's going on around us. Meditation, on the other hand, often involves techniques to focus the mind, achieve a mentally clear and emotionally calm state. Both practices have been shown to reduce stress hormones and lower blood pressure.

- **Deep Breathing Exercises:** Deep breathing is a simple yet effective way to reduce stress. Techniques like diaphragmatic breathing, where you breathe deeply into the belly rather than shallowly into the chest, can activate the body's relaxation response, reducing stress hormone levels, decreasing heart rate, and lowering blood pressure.

- **Regular Physical Activity:** Exercise is a well-known stress reliever. Activities like walking, jogging, swimming, cycling, yoga, and tai chi not only improve physical health but also boost endorphins, the body's natural mood elevators. Yoga and tai chi, in particular, combine physical movement with mindfulness and deep breathing, making them excellent choices for stress reduction.

- **Adequate Social Support:** A strong social network provides emotional support, which is crucial for managing stress. Talking with friends and family, participating in group activities, and even seeking professional help can provide relief from stress. Feeling connected and supported reduces feelings of loneliness and anxiety, which can exacerbate stress.

## Developing a Stress Management Routine

To effectively manage stress, it's important to identify personal stress triggers and develop a routine that incorporates stress-reduction techniques. This might involve setting aside time each day for mindfulness or meditation, engaging in regular physical activity, or reaching out to friends and family for social interaction. Even small changes, like practicing a few minutes of deep breathing when feeling overwhelmed, can make a significant difference in managing stress levels.

## Additional Strategies for Stress Management

- **Time Management:** Learning to prioritize tasks and manage time effectively can reduce the feeling of being overwhelmed, a common stressor.
- **Healthy Eating Habits:** Maintaining a balanced diet, like the DASH Diet, can provide the

necessary nutrients to support the body during stressful times.

- **Quality Sleep:** Adequate sleep is crucial for stress management. Establishing a regular sleep schedule and creating a restful environment can improve sleep quality.

## Importance of Sleep and Hydration in Heart Health

The role of sleep and hydration in maintaining heart health is pivotal yet often underestimated. They are crucial components of a holistic approach to health, complementing dietary and exercise habits, such as those advocated by the DASH Diet.

### The Role of Sleep in Heart Health

Quality sleep plays a significant role in heart health. It's during sleep that the body undergoes repair and regeneration processes essential for cardiovascular health. Poor sleep quality or insufficient sleep duration is linked to various heart-related issues:

- **Increased Blood Pressure:** Lack of sleep can cause disruptions in the body's natural circadian rhythms, leading to increased blood pressure, a major risk factor for heart disease.

- **Elevated Stress Hormones:** Insufficient sleep can elevate cortisol levels, the stress hormone, which in turn can strain the heart.

- **Impact on Metabolism:** Poor sleep patterns can affect the body's metabolism, increasing the risk of obesity, diabetes, and subsequently, heart disease.

**Tips for Better Sleep**

To improve sleep quality and duration, consider the following strategies:

- **Consistent Sleep Schedule:** Regularity in sleep patterns helps to synchronize the body's internal clock, improving sleep quality. Going to bed and waking up at the same time every day, including weekends, helps establish a consistent rhythm.

- **Create a Sleep-Inducing Environment:** A tranquil, dark, and cool environment can significantly enhance the quality of sleep. Using blackout curtains, eye masks, and maintaining a comfortable temperature can create conducive conditions for restful sleep.

- **Limit Exposure to Screens Before Bedtime:** Electronic devices emit blue light, which can interfere with the production of melatonin, the sleep hormone. Reducing screen time at least an hour before bedtime can help in maintaining the natural sleep-wake cycle.

- **Relaxation Techniques:** Activities like reading a book, taking a warm bath, practicing gentle yoga, or meditation can be effective in calming the mind and preparing the body for sleep. These practices reduce stress and promote relaxation, making it easier to fall asleep.

## The Importance of Hydration

Hydration is a critical yet often overlooked component of heart health. Proper hydration supports the heart's function in several ways:

- **Efficient Blood Circulation:** Adequate hydration aids in maintaining the blood's viscosity, making it easier for the heart to pump.

- **Muscle Function:** Water is essential for muscle function, including the heart muscle. Dehydration can lead to muscle fatigue, impacting heart health.

- **Digestion of Nutrients:** Water plays a vital role in the digestion and absorption of nutrients from the food, essential for overall health, including the heart.

## Tips for Staying Hydrated

To ensure proper hydration, follow these tips:

- **Drink Plenty of Water:** The general recommendation is to drink at least 8-10 glasses of water per day. However, individual needs may vary depending on factors like climate, exercise intensity, and overall health.

- **Incorporate Foods with High Water Content:** Consuming fruits and vegetables with high water content, such as cucumbers, tomatoes, oranges, and watermelon, can contribute to overall hydration. These foods also provide essential nutrients and fiber.

- **Monitor Hydration Levels:** Be aware of the signs of dehydration, which include dark-colored urine, dry mouth, fatigue, and dizziness. Monitoring these signs can help in maintaining adequate hydration levels.

- **Avoid Excessive Caffeine and Alcohol:** These can act as diuretics, leading to increased fluid loss. Moderating the intake of beverages like coffee and alcohol can help maintain hydration levels.

# CHAPTER 7

# OVERCOMING CHALLENGES

## Dealing with Dietary Restrictions and Allergies

Navigating dietary restrictions and allergies while adhering to the DASH Diet can indeed be a challenging aspect for many. This diet, which focuses on reducing hypertension and improving heart health, primarily emphasizes the intake of fruits, vegetables, whole grains, and lean proteins. However, for individuals with specific food allergies or intolerances, this can pose unique challenges that require careful consideration and adaptation.

## 1. Understanding Personal Restrictions

The first and foremost step in this journey is to have a clear understanding of one's personal dietary restrictions. Allergies and intolerances vary widely, and what might be a healthy option for one individual could be harmful to another. For example, if you are lactose intolerant, the DASH Diet's recommendation for low-fat dairy products might not be suitable for you. In such cases, finding alternatives becomes essential. Lactose-free milk or plant-based alternatives such as almond, soy, or oat milk can be excellent substitutes. These options allow you to enjoy the benefits of dairy - such as calcium and vitamin D - without the adverse effects of lactose.

For individuals with gluten sensitivity or celiac disease, the emphasis on whole grains in the DASH Diet can be another area of concern. Fortunately, there are numerous gluten-free whole grain options available, such as quinoa, brown rice, and buckwheat. These grains offer the same heart-healthy benefits without the gluten.

## 2. Customizing Your Diet Plan

The flexibility of the DASH Diet is one of its greatest strengths. It's not a rigid plan but rather a set of guidelines that can be adjusted according to individual needs and preferences. If you have a nut allergy, for instance, the common recommendation to consume nuts for healthy fats and proteins needs rethinking. In such cases, seeds like flaxseeds, chia seeds, or pumpkin seeds can be excellent alternatives. They are not only safe for those with nut allergies but also rich in omega-3 fatty acids and fiber.

Customization also extends to how you prepare your meals. For instance, if you're allergic to certain spices that are commonly used in DASH Diet recipes, you can experiment with other herbs and spices that don't trigger your allergies. The goal is to make the diet work for you, not against you.

## 3. Seeking Professional Advice

Despite your best efforts, aligning the DASH Diet with complex dietary restrictions can sometimes be daunting. This is where professional advice becomes invaluable. A registered dietitian or a nutritionist can offer personalized guidance, ensuring that you adhere to the DASH Diet's principles without compromising your health.

A dietitian can help you navigate the intricacies of your dietary restrictions, suggest alternative food options, and even help in meal planning. They can ensure that your modified DASH Diet plan is nutritionally balanced and caters to your specific health needs. This professional guidance can be particularly crucial for those with multiple or severe allergies, as they require more intricate diet modifications.

# Budget-Friendly Tips for the DASH Diet

Following a healthy diet like the DASH Diet often comes with the misconception that it is inherently expensive. Many people associate healthy eating with high-cost organic produce or specialty health foods. However, adhering to the DASH Diet does not have to strain your wallet. With some smart strategies and planning, you can enjoy the health benefits of this diet without overspending. Let's delve deeper into these budget-friendly tips:

## 1. Plan Your Meals

Strategic Meal Planning: Begin each week with a solid meal plan. This means deciding in advance what you'll eat for each meal, including snacks. By planning, you can build meals around ingredients you already have, reducing waste.

- **Shopping List Is Key:** Once your meals are planned, create a shopping list. Stick to this list when you shop to avoid impulse purchases, which often tend to be unnecessary and more expensive items.

- **Batch Cooking and Leftovers:** Consider preparing meals in batches. This approach not only saves time but also ingredients. Leftovers can be repurposed into new meals, ensuring nothing goes to waste.

## 2. Buy In-Season Produce

- **Explore Local Farmers Markets:** Farmers markets can be a great source for fresh, in-season produce. Prices are often lower than in supermarkets, and you're supporting local farmers.

- **Stay Informed About Seasonal Produce:** Knowing what fruits and vegetables are in season helps in planning your meals around more affordable, yet nutritious options. For instance, berries are cheaper in summer, while squash is more budget-friendly in the fall.

## 3. Opt for Frozen or Canned Options

- **Frozen Goods Are Your Friends:** Frozen fruits and vegetables are picked and frozen at their peak, so they retain most of their nutrients. They're a great alternative, especially for out-of-season produce.

- **Choose Canned Foods Wisely:** When selecting canned goods, look for options that say "no added salt" or "no added sugar." This ensures you're sticking to the DASH Diet's low-sodium, low-sugar principles.

- **Diverse Uses:** Frozen and canned goods are incredibly versatile. They can be used in a variety of dishes, from stir-fries to smoothies, making them convenient and cost-effective.

## 4. Embrace Whole Grains in Bulk

- **Bulk Buying Benefits:** Purchasing whole grains in bulk is generally cheaper than buying smaller, packaged quantities. Store them properly to extend their shelf life.

- **Versatility in Meals:** Whole grains like brown rice and quinoa can be used in multiple meals throughout the week – from a side dish to a salad base or even in soups.

## 5. Cook at Home

- **Home Cooking Economies:** Cooking at home is usually much more economical than dining out or buying pre-made meals. It also gives you complete control over what goes into your food, which is essential for adhering to the DASH Diet.

- **Prep in Advance:** Utilize meal prep techniques. Preparing ingredients ahead of time makes it easier to stick to your meal plan during a busy week.

- **Learn and Experiment:** Cooking at home can be a fun and rewarding experience. Experiment with new recipes and flavors to keep your meals interesting and enjoyable.

## 6. Additional Tips

- **Use Coupons and Discounts:** Keep an eye out for coupons, discounts, and sales at your local grocery stores. Many stores offer loyalty programs that can provide substantial savings over time.

- **Reduce Meat Consumption:** Meat can be one of the more expensive items in your grocery budget.

Consider reducing meat consumption and substituting with other protein sources like beans and lentils, which are staples in the DASH Diet and are more budget-friendly.

- **Grow Your Own:** If possible, start a small vegetable garden. Growing your own produce can be a cost-effective and rewarding way to ensure a supply of fresh ingredients.

- **Community Resources:** Look into community-supported agriculture (CSA) programs or co-ops in your area. These can offer fresh produce at lower prices and are a great way to support local farmers.

## Staying Motivated and Managing Setbacks

Staying motivated and managing setbacks is perhaps the most crucial part of adhering to the DASH Diet. Change is never easy, and it's normal to face hurdles along the way.

1. **Set Realistic Goals:** Instead of aiming for quick, dramatic changes, set achievable goals. For instance, start by incorporating

more vegetables into your meals or reducing your sodium intake gradually.

2.  **Track Your Progress:** Keep a food diary or use a health app to track your progress. Monitoring your journey not only helps in staying on course but also provides a sense of accomplishment.

3.  **Find Support:** Whether it's a dietitian, a support group, or family and friends, having a support system can make a significant difference. Sharing your goals, struggles, and successes with others can provide motivation and accountability.

4.  **Celebrate Small Wins:** Every step in the right direction is a win. Celebrated these moments. Whether it's choosing a healthy snack over a sugary one or seeing an improvement in your blood pressure, acknowledging these victories can boost your motivation.

5.  **Be Kind to Yourself:** Setbacks are a normal part of any journey. If you find

yourself straying from the diet, don't be too hard on yourself. Reflect on what led to the setback and plan on how to avoid it in the future.

6.  **Keep Learning:** The more you know about the DASH Diet and heart health, the more empowered you'll feel. Keep educating yourself. The understanding of why certain foods are better choices reinforces the commitment to those choices.

7.  **Adjust and Adapt:** Flexibility is key. If a certain aspect of the diet isn't working for you, be willing to adjust and adapt. The DASH Diet is not one-size-fits-all, and it's okay to tweak it to fit your lifestyle and preferences.

# CHAPTER 8

# LATEST RESEARCH AND DEVELOPMENTS IN HEART HEALTH AND THE DASH DIET

The field of nutrition and heart health is continuously evolving, with new studies and innovations constantly reshaping our understanding of what it means to eat healthily, particularly concerning the DASH (Dietary Approaches to Stop Hypertension) Diet. This diet, initially designed to combat high blood pressure, has since been recognized for its broader benefits in promoting heart health. In this comprehensive exploration, we delve into the latest research and developments surrounding the DASH Diet and general heart health nutrition.

## Recent Studies on the DASH Diet

1. **Expanded Benefits Beyond Blood Pressure:** Recent studies have extended the known benefits of the DASH Diet beyond just lowering blood pressure. Research has indicated its effectiveness in reducing the risk of heart disease, stroke, and even certain types of cancer. For instance, a study published in the 'Journal of the American Heart Association' found

that adherence to the DASH Diet was associated with a lower risk of heart failure in people under 75.

2. **Impact on Kidney Health:** The DASH Diet's positive effects on kidney health have been a focal point in recent research. A study in the 'American Journal of Kidney Diseases' highlighted that following the DASH Diet could help in the prevention of kidney stones, owing to its emphasis on fruits, vegetables, and low dairy intake.

3. **Cognitive Benefits:** Emerging research has also begun to explore the cognitive benefits associated with the DASH Diet. A study in 'Neurology' suggested that the diet might slow the rate of cognitive decline in stroke survivors. This is attributed to the diet's high content of nutrients that are beneficial for brain health.

4. **Effectiveness in Weight Loss:** While the DASH Diet was not originally designed for weight loss, recent studies have shown it can be effective in this regard when combined with reduced calorie intake. Research in the 'Journal of Nutrition' demonstrated that participants following a calorie-restricted DASH

Diet experienced significant weight loss and reduction in body fat.

5.  **Improved Heart Health Markers:** A critical area of recent study is the diet's impact on overall heart health markers, including cholesterol and blood sugar levels. Research indicates that the DASH Diet can improve these markers, further lowering the risk of heart disease.

## Innovations in Heart Health Nutrition

1.  **Personalized Nutrition Plans:** One of the most significant advancements in heart health nutrition is the shift towards personalized diet plans. Advances in genetic testing and biotechnology have made it possible to tailor dietary recommendations based on individual genetic profiles, lifestyle, and health conditions. This personalized approach can optimize the effectiveness of diets like DASH for individual needs.

2.  **Plant-based Variations of the DASH Diet:** The rise of plant-based eating has led to innovations in the DASH Diet, with variations that emphasize vegetarian and vegan options. These plant-based

versions focus on fruits, vegetables, nuts, seeds, and legumes, aligning with the principles of the DASH Diet while catering to those following a plant-based lifestyle.

3. **Integration of Technology in Diet Planning:** Technology plays a crucial role in modern heart health nutrition. Mobile apps and online platforms now offer personalized tracking of dietary intake, making it easier for individuals to adhere to diets like the DASH Diet. These tools often include features for monitoring blood pressure and other health metrics, providing a comprehensive approach to heart health.

4. **The Role of Gut Health:** Recent studies have highlighted the importance of gut health in overall cardiovascular wellness. Probiotics and prebiotics are being increasingly recognized for their role in heart health, leading to dietary recommendations that include fermented foods and fiber-rich ingredients, complementing the principles of the DASH Diet.

5. **Anti-Inflammatory Foods:** There is a growing focus on anti-inflammatory foods in heart health nutrition. Chronic inflammation is a known risk factor for heart

disease, and diets rich in anti-inflammatory foods like omega-3 fatty acids, found in fish, flaxseeds, and walnuts, are being recommended alongside the DASH Diet principles.

# CONCLUSION

The DASH (Dietary Approaches to Stop Hypertension) Diet, initially developed to combat hypertension, has emerged as a multi-faceted nutritional strategy with far-reaching benefits for heart health and beyond. This conclusion consolidates the extensive discussion on the DASH Diet, highlighting its key aspects, recent research findings, and expanded health benefits.

**Core Elements of the DASH Diet:** The diet emphasizes whole grains, fruits, vegetables, lean proteins, and low-fat dairy, focusing on nutrient-rich foods while limiting sodium, saturated fats, and sugars. It promotes a balanced intake of foods that are essential for maintaining healthy blood pressure levels and overall cardiovascular health.

**Expanded Benefits Beyond Blood Pressure Control:** Recent studies have significantly broadened the DASH Diet's impact. It is now recognized for its effectiveness in reducing the risk of heart disease, stroke, and certain types of cancer. Notably, it has also been linked with the prevention of mild mental impairments, which can be a precursor to dementia. A 2023 study highlighted the diet's dramatic effects in lowering the risk of heart problems, particularly in women and Black adults. Additionally, it has been associated with a lower risk of cognitive decline among women over 40.

**Impact on Kidney Health:** Research from Johns Hopkins University revealed that adherence to the DASH Diet significantly reduces the risk of developing chronic kidney disease. The diet's preventive role against kidney disease is attributed to its effectiveness in lowering blood pressure and reducing dietary acid load.

**Effectiveness in Weight Loss and Metabolic Health:** While not originally designed for weight loss, the DASH Diet has been effective in this area when combined with reduced calorie intake. Studies involving obese patients with non-alcoholic fatty liver disease (NAFLD) showed that the diet could significantly improve weight, glycemia, inflammation, and liver function.

**Improved Heart Health Markers:** The diet has been shown to lower LDL cholesterol (the "bad" cholesterol), a major risk factor for cardiovascular disease. Additionally, a study in the Journal of the American College of Cardiology linked the DASH Diet with a reduction in heart damage.

*The DASH Diet stands as a comprehensive dietary approach, offering a multitude of health benefits beyond its original purpose of lowering blood pressure. Its principles of emphasizing whole, nutrient-rich foods and limiting harmful components align with the broader goals of promoting heart health, preventing chronic diseases, and improving overall well-being. The expanding body of research underscores its potential as a holistic dietary strategy, making it a valuable tool for individuals seeking to improve their health and reduce the risk of various health conditions. As such, the DASH Diet not only addresses specific health concerns like hypertension and heart disease but also serves as a foundation for a healthier, more balanced lifestyle.*